Nursing Research—Mistakes and Misconceptions

Nursing Research—
Mistakes and Misconceptions

A light-hearted personal account of things that did or could go wrong

Lisbeth Hockey OBE

SRN HV QNS PhD FRCN HonFRCGP

Formerly Director, Nursing Research Unit, University of Edinburgh

CHURCHILL LIVINGSTONE

EDINBURGH LONDON MELBOURNE AND NEW YORK 1985

CHURCHILL LIVINGSTONE
Medical Division of Longman Group Limited

Distributed in the United States of America by
Churchill Livingstone Inc., 1560 Broadway, New York,
N.Y. 10036, and by associated companies, branches
and representatives throughout the world.

First published 1985

ISBN 0 443 02862 1

British Library Cataloguing in Publication Data
Hockey, Lisbeth
Nursing research—mistakes and misconceptions.
1. Nursing Research
I. Title
610.73'072 RT81.5

Library of Congress Cataloguing in Publication Data
Hockey, Lisbeth.
Nursing research, mistakes and misconceptions.
1. Nursing—Research—miscellanea. I. Title.
[DNLM: 1. Nursing. 2. Research—methods. WY 20.5 H685n]
RT81.5.H63 1985 610.73'072 84-12055

Printed in Hong Kong
by Wing Lee Printing Co Ltd

Preface

I came into research about 25 years ago and almost by chance. I had many misconceptions about research to start with and 25 years is a long period in which to make mistakes. There were many times when I said to myself: 'I wish someone had told me...'. So, I decided to jot down some of the things that actually or nearly went wrong, things that I could have been alerted to. Over the years I accumulated quite a lot of such jottings and the purpose of this little book is to warn others of things that I would have liked to be warned about myself. It may not work, perhaps we learn most from our own mistakes which can so easily be made. Watch, beware!

The book is divided into eight chapters followed by a brief epilogue. Each chapter relates one or more actual situations in which I found myself and each illustrates specific mistakes or misconceptions. The specific incidents illustrate more general issues which tend to confront researchers over and over again. Therefore, each chapter concludes with the lessons that could be learned from it; it is *hindsight advice* and I can say, with some conviction, that hindsight is more reliable than foresight—at least most of the time.

Edinburgh 1985   L.H.

Acknowledgements

First, I would like to record sincere thanks to my main research 'mentor', Miss H. Marjorie Simpson, who helped me to see and put right some of my many mistakes. She was one of the founder members of the early Nursing Research Discussion Group all of whom provided important support.

The late Miss Alice Thompson, former librarian of the Royal College of Nursing, helped me to find my way around a library and to use it with benefit.

Without my employers and sponsors I would not have had the opportunity for research and the enjoyment and experience gained from it. I could not have learned from my mistakes.

Over the years many people criticized my work and, in retrospect, I am grateful to most of them.

In the production of this small book I was helped by the encouragement of many friends, colleagues and students who thought it was a good idea. Special thanks are due to the staff of Churchill Livingstone for their interest and constructive suggestions.

Dr Albert Pilliner kindly read the draft and made most helpful comments. Mrs Muriel Armstrong typed the manuscript in record time.

L.H.

Contents

Contents

Introduction

If I had no jottings to resort to it would be difficult to envisage what it was like 25–40 years ago when I first began to think about nursing research. Even more difficult is it to believe my own naivety in the early stages of my nursing career, about 45 years ago. Although memory helps me to re-live some of the more profound experiences most vividly, I know what tricks memory can play and hope that my notes, however sketchy, have kept me a great deal closer to the truth.

My first note is dated September 1940 and relates the elements of a discussion between a ward sister and myself, then a very junior 'probationer nurse'. I was concerned about some patients getting bedsores (remember it was 1940, long before pressure sores took over) and others did not: 'It could be the bed linen—it feels like boards, but that is the same for *all* patients.' The ward sister did not seem too pleased. She informed me that I was here to heal the sores not to ask questions about them, that we were far too busy, and in any case, if we knew the answer there wouldn't be any sores.

I wrote: 'We don't know the answer, but shouldn't we?'

A further 3 years passed before my next note: 'Here

we are, years later, no questions asked and none answered; but there is a war on, not the best time for question asking. It takes us all every ounce of energy just to keep going.'

Fever nursing in London during the 'Blitz' was not exactly fun. Some patients were nursed in cubicles with glass partitions between them to 'prevent cross infection'. As a result of the bombing and the risk of injury from shattered glass, the glass partitions were removed. We did *not* get any cross infection. Why not, when the glass partitions had been sacrosanct in preventing it? 'Why, Sister, don't we? What is preventing it now?' The Sister told me that I was tempting providence. 'Keep washing your hands,' she advised. 'Watch and pray. We don't know why not, but we are thankful.'

My note says: 'We don't know why not, but shouldn't we?'

At that time it seemed that nothing could be done to get answers to simple and fundamental questions. Yet, having come to nursing from another better established discipline I had a nagging feeling that there *should* be scientific answers to both questions and to many others. Scientific answers? What has science got to do with nursing? Not much at that time, that was certain, but it is different now!

It was not until a small number of nurses initiated a Research Discussion Group that the possibility of nursing research came into my thinking. Then the idea took over, way beyond all reason. I thought that research would very soon provide answers to all questions. I was annoyed with myself for not having realized much earlier the potential of research.

I wrote: 'Thank God for some nurses with imagination and guts; now we must make up for lost time.'

That was about 30 years ago.

When I began my research activity the resources in terms of relevant literature were extremely sparse. The nurse researcher of today is much better off. The bibliography at the end of this book represents a small selection of useful texts, each of which has its own reference list taking the reader further.

Through sharing the mistakes I made, I hope to say '*Don't!*' Through presenting a bibliography on various aspects of research methodology, I hope to say '*Do!*'

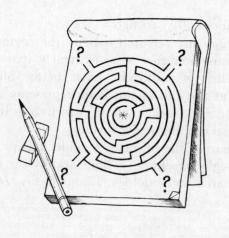

One
Fantasies about what research can do

Research sounds great and from never having entered
nursing thinking at all, it has become almost a cliché.
It has certainly taken off impressively in the last 30
years. However, when I first became involved I had
weird and wonderful ideas about what research might
achieve.

My first opportunity came when I was working at
the headquarters of the district nursing service and the
procedures used by district nursing staff for the
sterilization of equipment were being called into
question. No problem, I thought naively, we'll do some
research.

At that time I was working with a non-nurse
graduate who not only had a better idea of research
than me which was not too difficult—but who also
asked extremely pertinent questions about matters
which we, as nurses, took for granted and could not
explain. My research question was: 'Are the
sterilization procedures, as carried out by district
nurses, safe?' My idea was to go out and see what they
were doing, just a couple of weeks' observation would
provide the answer.

My colleague was clearly extremely doubtful and
asked: 'What is safe practice? Which nurses will you go

5

out to watch? Will they behave normally when they are being watched or will they try to please you? Which specific procedures will you watch? Are all homes equally easy or difficult to work in? How will you prove your point at the end?'

Those were just some of her questions and, of course, I could answer hardly any of them. One of my jottings indicates annoyance at her apparent 'arrogance': 'Just because she is a graduate she thinks she knows it all.' Much later I wrote 'What a lot of things we just accept without questioning; here we are again. She asked sensible questions and saved the research. I should have been more tolerant, indeed grateful, for having been helped to think.'

My idea of getting the answer to my research question in a few weeks was soon squashed; it could not be done like that; it required a complex research design, a carefully conducted data collection and analysis. Above all, it needed clear definitions of what was wanted. All this happened eventually but it took sweat and tears, in addition to money. Even then, many loose ends were left and many more questions were raised than were answered. That study taught me a great deal but some fantasies remained.

While still working at the same place I was asked to organize district nurse training in London. It was patchy and needed co-ordination. The training was based on a syllabus devised by my employers in collaboration with senior community nursing staff. It was a 'sacred' syllabus and had been used for many years.

The task I was given, prompted me to ask whether

the syllabus was (still) appropriate; did it prepare district nurses for the work expected of them when they were qualified? I voiced the question and was told in no uncertain manner that the syllabus was perfectly good enough for hundreds of nurses and who was I to question it. However, I was given permission to do a 'simple survey' if it would make me happy: 'Good, research will give the answer.'

Of course, I remembered that I needed to define my terms. In the previous study I had been caught out by 'safe practice'; this time it was 'appropriate preparation'. Who should say it is appropriate and how does one link the training with the work? Is not every situation different? I decided that we could ask the district nurses themselves if they considered their training appropriate and we could also watch them at work. I tried it out on a few of them but, being a bit of a cynic, I became suspicious about their completely positive comments on their training. Perhaps they just refused to criticize their training; moreover, could they really be expected to remember if their current knowledge and skills came from training or from their experience afterwards?

It was finally decided that we needed to find out first of all what district nursing is. If we don't know what district nursing consists of, how can we prepare nurses appropriately for it? So, let us watch district nurses at work and we did. The nurses washed patients; they made beds; they applied dressings to wounds, mostly to ulcerated legs; they made cups of tea; they helped patients to walk; they fetched prescriptions from the doctor's surgery and medicaments from the chemist, etc., etc. The list of jobs performed by district nurses was studied—surely, not all of those activities are 'nursing'? They are non-nursing duties; but we *watched* district nurses in order to find out what district nursing *is* and then we did not like the findings. So, can research tell us what district nursing *is*?

It obviously can *not* give us this information *if* it is possible for district nursing to be something different from what district nurses do. The questions 'What is district nursing?' or, indeed, 'What is nursing?' are not the kind of questions which are amenable to research. I learned it the hard way. Research can tell us what nurses do and we can then decide which, if any, of the activities undertaken by nurses should be called nursing. Alternatively, we can make a policy decision about what nursing *should* be and then find out, through one of many procedures available to researchers, whether the work nurses actually do reflects the policy decision or not.

Where does this leave us if we want to know if our policy decision was wise, if what we decreed nurses should do is appropriate in meeting patients' needs—a term we use all too freely? What *are* patients' needs?

'Can research tell us what the needs of patients are. Yes or no?'

I'm afraid the answer must be 'no'. This is yet another question which, in its present form, is *not* a researchable question.

Hindsight advice

1. Probably the most important lesson is that although we

should persist in asking questions, not all questions are researchable. Some questions are matters for policy decisions and not for research; others have to be re-formulated to make them researchable.

2. All terms must be clearly defined; my examples were 'safe practice' and 'appropriate training'. There are many, many other terms in nursing which are used regularly in spite of obvious ambiguities. My jottings show that I had problems with 'surgical' patients and with 'terminal' care. My colleagues told me that they knew what was meant but could not define it. 'Good nursing' is another favourite.

3. Research is a scientific process and it takes time. People who want answers to complex research questions by 'tomorrow' are misguided. Research requires not only time but also other resources, such as finance and expertise. What a dreadful mess I would have made of my early studies if I had not had the benefit of a level-headed, clear-thinking colleague, and a peer group of early nurse researchers with whom one could be really honest and who gave one the courage to tell employers that their expectations were unrealistic.

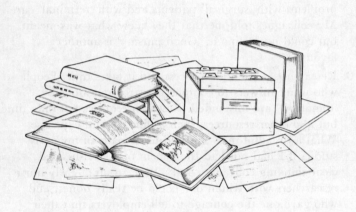

Two
Misconceptions about how to do research

As I indicated in Chapter One, I did eventually discover that research involved a scientific process which required 'know-how'. However, it was not too easy for me to accept that I did not possess this 'know-how', especially as my employers seemed to think that I could mount a survey without any help from anyone. In the beginning, their idea as well as mine was 'just to go and find out'. Fortunately, I have always enjoyed browsing in libraries and, even more fortunately, there was the Research Discussion Group to which I referred in the Introduction. Research is about 'finding out', but it is not quite as simple as I imagined it to be; although the literature and my friends helped me, I still blundered with great vigour.

My jotting, dated January 1964, says: 'I must ask the district nurses how they get on with the General Practitioners (GPs) whose patients they are nursing. Then I'll ask the GPs about the nurses; that shouldn't really be too difficult and no-one can argue about things which are quoted straight from the horse's mouth. I'll send them a polite letter and see what happens.' Apparently, although it is hard to believe now, I must have done just that but, thankfully, I learned from my stupidity before going too far.

Just 2 months later, I wrote: 'How could I have been so naive? Here I am with some rude answers from GPs, one implying that he had better things to do than write novels about the nurses he rarely saw anyway; another, sending me seven pages of heart-rending instances where nurses could have helped him but didn't and telling me how he would run a district nursing service if he were given the chance. A nurse wrote to say that she doesn't know the GPs and, in any case, she would never talk about them; 'it was not professional'. There were others. What was I to do?

What is the research process and how does one set about it?

I knew all about the need to have definitions, but how do you define a 'good relationship with GPs or district nurses?' It leaves the way wide open for quite embarrassing misinterpretations. I took the problem to my research colleagues who, even at that time, were still only a small group of committed pioneers who met monthly in each other's homes. I had to wait my turn; they were understanding and supportive and we learned a great deal from each other.

They asked me what my 'research question' was— simply 'How do district nurses and GPs get on with each other?' When they asked what information I would need for an answer to this question, I had no clear plan. I had vague half-baked ideas which needed to be sharpened and refined. They asked me if I had searched the literature to see if anyone else had done a similar study. I did not really like to confess (a) that I didn't quite know what they meant by 'searching the literature', (b) that I certainly had not done whatever it was, and (c) that I had no idea how to set about it anyway.

My note says: 'Now I am really stuck; why didn't I ask? Pride will not get you anywhere. How do you "search the literature"? I do wish someone could just tell me not only how, but also why? If someone else has done my project I don't really want anyone to know about it because *I* want to do it. It interests me.'

Fortunately, commonsense, meagre as it seemed to be, intervened and I sneaked into the library of the Royal College of Nursing and searched with the help of the long-suffering and extremely helpful librarian.* She explained to me why it was necessary to do such a search and I pass her advice on to the readers of this little book. First, she said, it is unwise to dabble in an area of which you know very little (she was always refreshingly honest and forthright); second, it would be a pity not to know about the pitfalls someone else might have encountered which would help you to avoid them; third, no-one else's study would have been so large that it could not do with being done again in your area; and, lastly, if you use a questionnaire similar to that of the other person whom you may find in your search, you may be able to compare your results.

So, translating her very early amazingly insightful advice into more up-to-date technical terms, she said that one must become familiar with the area of one's intended research by reading about it as much as possible, that one should attempt to avoid the mistakes

*The late Miss Alice Thompson who pioneered the valuable Nursing Bibliography.

that other people made (which, incidentally, is the main purpose of this book), that small studies could be made more useful in terms of application and generalizability if they were replicated and that the use of tools already validated by other researchers would not only ease the research process but would also make it possible for findings to be compared. These were matters I had never given any thought to before and they were, and continue to be, matters of extreme importance.

With her help, I searched the literature, which taught me how to use a library; although I had always enjoyed browsing, I had never been systematic about it. Of course, there were many times when I got side-tracked from my main intended path and had to steer myself back on course.

I discovered literature in the library that I had never even heard about before: historical material, biographies of famous nurses, government reports and dozens of journals with absorbing contents. Over and over again I found myself reading articles which had nothing at all to do with my research topic, and closing time came without much relevant 'searching' having been done. My available time was limited and I became frantic, often being near to giving up.

It seemed improbable to me that there was no more literature on my subject matter than I found; there seemed to be an abundance of every other subject except mine. When I mentioned my concern to the Research Discussion Group, my friends reassured me. They had not come across much, if any, research on district nursing in general and no-one had even heard of anyone wishing to explore inter-professional relationships. My note says: 'I asked them if a study looking at the relationships between GPs and district nurses constituted "virgin territory" and they burst into hysterical laughing; maybe it was an unfortunate way of putting it! I don't feel like laughing though, I need help.'

Looking back on my library work I learned a great deal although I only found a few legislation extracts and Working Party Reports which were in any way relevant for me at that time. I scribbled them out on pieces of paper which I thought I had put in my research folder. When the time came to refer to them they were nowhere to be found and precious hours were wasted searching not the literature but my desk, my handbags, my brief case, my books, my everything. Eventually, they all came to light but my troubles were far from over.

There were two references I wanted to look at again but, alas, my rough piece of paper did not tell me in which volume of a specific journal I had read one of them, which meant starting to look for it all over again. The other referrence came from a book; I had the title of the book, its author and its publisher—so far, so good! I managed to obtain the book after it had to be recalled from another borrower; it was a tome. My jotting says: 'You really are stupid—how did you think you could ever find this again in a book of 470 pages? You should have noted the page number; write this down quickly so you can tell others how important it is.' I mentioned it to my friend who had already written a thesis. 'Oh dear, I am so sorry I didn't warn you, 'she sympathized.' I had a similar problem and I didn't know that one must give page numbers in the reference list for a thesis. I wasted hours of time and was at the point of suicide.'

As this small book is intended to be really honest I must confess that I omitted the page numbers of some of my references in reports I had published. It was a mistake to do that; a reference list should enable an interested reader to find the references; all I did was to transfer the chore of chasing an obscure reference to the poor reader.

Don't do as I did; I am not proud of it.

I devoted a large part of this chapter to the literature search which is only one part, though a most important one, of the research process. What about the next stages?

When I started, I had little idea of what should happen next. In my case, the literature did not give me a great deal of help, simply because there had been no research on the topic I was interested in. It was a matter of starting from scratch. Of course, I asked around and people gave advice. My jotting says: 'People are really kind and helpful, but they all seem to suggest different ways of tackling the job. How do I know which to take?'

By that time, I had found an evening course at the University of London which offered statistics for beginners. The effort of attending it after a hard day's work was enormous, especially as it all sounded totally confusing at first, but I can honestly say, it was worth every bit of it. Most important, I found another student who was interested in my problems and helped me to talk them through. Once again, I was challenged to re-phrase my research question and to write down what information I needed and from whom, in order to answer it.

My fellow student, a non-nurse sociologist, explained that each research question needed a different kind of approach depending on its nature. He also told me that you should try out your method by doing a pre-run of the study, a pilot study.

My note reads: 'I'll do a pilot study my way and we'll see what happens.'

It was 6 months later when I carried out the pilot study! 'The district nurses came in and answered all my questions without a problem. They seemed quite interested and they appreciated the tea and the book token we gave them for participating. So that is one part done. All I need to do is change a few questions around and explain to them what I mean by "working with GPs".' All the GPs who had been lecturing on the training courses received a questionnaire and all but two sent them back, that was six. They had mentioned no problems either.

I am sorry to confess that what I called a pilot study was just not good enough and the weaknesses soon came to light. Of course, both groups, the nurses and the GPs, were not typical of the total number. Using research terminology, they were not representative; the nurses were more interested than the average seemed to be; they were all working in South London so that they were close enough to come to see me; they were allowed to come in their duty time. The GPs had been involved in teaching and that made them different from the normal run of GPs. Some of them had been explaining how GPs and district nurses could work together more happily, so they had definite views about the topic. In my main study, things were very different indeed and many terms which had been used were not even understood. My study had not been clearly thought through and some of the answers I got, showed that I should have done a much better and more thorough pilot study.

I found a scribble in the margin of one of the returned questionnaires, *my* scribble, which said: 'She must have meant (1), so we'll code it that way. I can't think why she ticked (2). It is not clear though; maybe, the tick is meant to be for (1)?' I committed a serious mistake by guessing what I thought the person (the respondent) intended to indicate.

Don't do as I did; it starts you on a slippery slope which can be dangerous.

Further problems came with coding, with analysis and with writing up; they are discussed in other chapters. Suffice it to say here, that I should not have been allowed, still less encouraged, to undertake a study of this magnitude without much more help and guidance. My ideas of how to do research were absurdly naive and I had the most incredible misconceptions about it.

Hindsight advice

1. Do not neglect a thorough search of the literature. Ask the librarian if you need help. Keep a card index of all the references you think might be helpful later. Record every

detail about the source; don't forget the volume number of a journal and the page number of a book. To remember that you saw it in the top paragraph of a right hand page does *not* help!

2. Consult other people but decide when to stop getting advice. In many instances there are no totally right or totally wrong ways of proceeding; there are different ways. I found it helpful to set up a small Advisory Group of people who were really interested in the topic. Don't think that non-nurses have nothing to offer; their questions often help us to clarify our thoughts and challenge our assumptions.

3. Do not underestimate the importance of a *thorough* pilot study and do not tamper with the finally agreed questionnaire. Make sure that your pilot respondents represent the kind of people you want to include in your main study.

4. Use a clear way of showing the intended answer; a circle is safer than a tick:

    .... 3 ✓   .... ③
    4   4

5. Most important of all, remember that research requires some 'know-how' which you may not have. Don't let it stop you from pursuing your study, but be sure you get the kind of help you need.

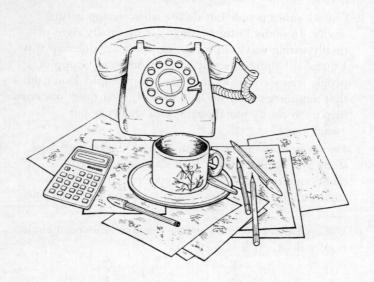

Three
Problems in taking off

I have not yet met a researcher who was not keen to get started. Some researchers, nurses and others, intend to do their research in order to get an academic qualification; others have to keep within the budget of a research grant; some may have both constraints, in terms of a time shortage. 'The later we get started, the later we'll finish' is an accepted statement which sounds as if it ought to be right, but I have found it not to be so in all cases. Sometimes, a delay in getting started helps to avoid hold-ups and complications later. The need for a thorough pilot study is mentioned in the preceding chapter. Clearly, the longer one spends on it, the longer will be the delay in getting started on the main study. However, the six completed questionnaires I had from a biased group of GPs were certainly not adequate to give me the all-clear for going ahead. I ran into trouble.

To start with, I needed a list of GPs to whom to send the final questionnaire and had not given much thought to where I might get it from. The district nursing staff in the areas I had selected for my study could give me the names and addresses of most, but not all, GPs. Understandably, they knew those with whom they came into contact but I wanted *all*. I tried various national and regional bodies including the British Medical Association (BMA), the Trades Union for the medical profession. After unbearable weeks of total silence I received a letter challenging the ethical implications of my proposed study and asking if I had been given permission by an Ethics Committee. The BMA had not heard about it before and they were somewhat indignant, to put it mildly. No, I had not taken my study to them for permission; why should I have done? I was not spending their money. I was not going to include any patients and I gave the GPs the chance to refuse to answer my questions. In my view it had nothing to do with the BMA; I only wanted their help in securing a list of GPs.

Nonetheless I was requested to take the study to the BMA Ethics Committee. The reasons given were that I was encroaching on a medical area, that GPs might not want to be approached and that the results of the study might have ethical implications. There was no way out of it and I had to wait patiently for another 6 weeks until the relevant committee had time on their agenda to discuss it. 'Why hadn't anyone told me that when I started? I could have saved so much time.' Eventually, the letter came giving approval but, alas, no list of GPs. Why didn't they tell me straight away that they 'do not divulge' members' addresses to anyone? Fair enough, but they could have said so much earlier.

In the end I found more appropriate sources for the information I needed but it took endless time. With the final questionnaire I sent a letter explaining the study and indicating (proudly) that it had been approved by the Ethics Committee of the BMA. This 'blessing' obviously did not melt the hearts of all GPs; two of them sent the blank forms back indicating that the BMA's consent put them off. I wrote: 'This is enough to make you give up for ever; how can one ever please everybody?'

Well one can't, but one should take obvious precautions and plan well ahead, building in the inevitable period of hiccoughs which seems to occur in most studies.

My list of GPs, or rather my many, many lists, arrived from various local sources and I was delighted until ... *until* I realized that many were on several lists and some, whom I knew to be practising in certain areas, were on none. I discovered that this was due to the fact that many GPs had more than one practice, often in different administrative areas, while many lived in one area but practised in another. What a muddle it all seemed to be and how much effort it took to sort it all out! In fact, we had to employ another research assistant, merely to draw up the final list of GPs on which each GP appeared once only and practised in one of the selected research areas. This list eventually constituted our 'sampling frame' but the task of drawing a random sample from it still remained. It was yet another important stage which looked so much simpler than it turned out to be.

Indeed, I was on the verge of making 'snap' decisions when it was pointed out to me, just in time, that the selection of my sample was absolutely crucial to the significance of the study and I needed statistical advice. By that time something like 10 weeks had passed and my frustration was as its highest. Fortunately, I got advice relatively quickly from a statistician who did not mind my stupid and naive questions. He was able to put me right and to help me throughout the study including the analysis stage.

He asked me, among other questions, what I would do if many GPs refused to co-operate. That possibility had not occurred to me; my 'pilot' GPs had been happy to help but, you will remember, they were not representative. 'Well,' I thought, 'we'll just have to rely on the ones who do see sense (how arrogant can you be!) and forget about the others.' 'But,' cautioned my statistical adviser, 'the ones who do complete your questionnaire may be as unrepresentative as your six pilot respondents were. You would not be able to place too much confidence in your findings, that is, if you want your study to be representative of all GPs in the areas from which you took your sample.' It became very clear to me that my preparations for 'take off' had been inadequate in a number of ways and that many of the problems I encountered could have been avoided.

In the course of our many discussions my statistical adviser asked me why I thought I needed whatever number of GPs and nurses I had decided on. It was just a good round number from which it seemed easy to calculate percentages—that was as far as my analysis was intended to go. He asked for an example of the kind of calculations I hoped to be able to make. I was delighted to share my hunch with him: 'For example.' I explained, 'I think that older GPs are less willing to admit that district nurses can think for themselves than younger GPs. So, I'll have a table showing GP age and their opinions about district nurses. I bet, the old ones

will be negative and the young ones positive.' I
remember him taking another slow and thorough look
at my draft questionnaire. Then, he looked at me in a
puzzled sort of way: 'How do you know the GPs age?'
Heavens, he was right! I had forgotten to include it
and, although it was not too late to insert it on the
final questionnaire, I had not tried the question out in
my pilot study. Therefore, I had no idea how GPs
would react to the question.

My jotting says: 'To-day I learned an important
lesson; one should really work out all one's calculations
from the pilot study and draw up mock tables. Had I
done that I would have realized that I had forgotten to
ask for the most important bit of information to prove
my point.' Reading this note now, I feel thoroughly
embarrassed that I had tried to do research in order to
'prove my point'—it was not a very objective approach
and I would advise strongly against it.

Having gone through so many hurdles in getting
research off the ground with a questionnaire and
interviewing schedule that had survived the heat of fire
in the form of committees, advisers, well-wisher etc. the
temptation to ask 'just a few' extra questions was too
great to be resisted. Of course, I did not break the rules
by changing a research tool that had been agreed;
nothing as grossly unethical as that. It was merely a
matter of sneaking in—at the very end, so as not to
change the sequence of the questions—some additional
topics. After all, when would I have another chance to
interview so many GPs or nurses? Surely, it was shrewd
to exploit the present situation by extracting from them
as much information as possible. It couldn't do any

harm. As I was solely responsible for all the interviews my seemingly innocent ploy did not involve anyone else.

It is true that the interviews took considerably longer than the time suggested when consent was first obtained but, so what? When respondents queried it, I gave them the opportunity to finish by saying: 'Of course, I quite understand that you have something else to do, but the information you are giving me is so important and no-one else is able to provide it for me. It will only take another ... minute or so.' In short, I used almost moral coercion and most of them seemed to accept it. However, what I had not realized then, as I do now, was that colleagues who wanted to get GPs to consent to research interviews in the area next to the one I had been working in, were not so happy. One said 'You say it will only take 20 minutes; but my partner who has a practice in ... had a similar request and he had to spend twice as long answering a whole lot of irrelevant questions; I just wouldn't have done it; I don't have the time.' She was able to get a 56% consent rate only and, although I don't know whether that was altogether my fault—in fact I doubt that it was—I worried about it.

The other, perhaps even more important, reason for not asking additional questions only in the interest of opportunism and possible further use of information is the dilemma I found myself in when it came to coding and processing those data. They just didn't fit in anywhere and I found it extremely hard to make any use of them either in that specific project or in any of my later work. I had collected information which was unnecessary, irrelevant and time-consuming for the respondent as well as for me as researcher; it also cost hard money in terms of computer time and analysis. I must say, it gave me a bad conscience and now I would not readily embark on or condone such an approach.

Hindsight advice

1. Make sure that your study is introduced to all the people who have a right to know about it and that it gets ethical approval from relevant committees, even if you cannot see the ethical implications yourself.
2. Do not start your main study until you have all plans for the field work totally completed, including contingency plans in the event of unexpected obstacles.
3. Enlist the help of a statistician at the very beginning of your work, even before the pilot study and try to find someone who does not mind helping the most pitiful ignoramus.
4. Build into your timetable a realistic margin for delays and use time delays in a positive way,such as more reading or extending pilot work, rather than getting impatient and agitated.
5. Do not start your main study until you have analysed your pilot study and have drawn up dummy tables, where appropriate of course (not every piece of research has tables). Dummy tables help in ensuring that you will have all the necessary information.
6. It is not wise to embark on research in order to 'prove one's point'. It may lead to dishonesty or disappointment. It should be done to get as closely as possible to the facts.
7. Do not ask questions 'just in case' they come in useful.

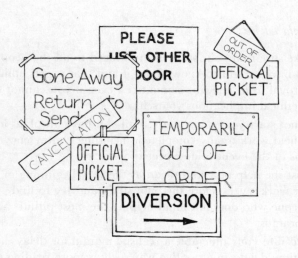

Four
When good plans can go wrong

This is a short chapter just to warn those who believe that all their preparations are made and that it is quite impossible for anything to go wrong. Let me tell you, it can, it usually does and it helps to know that it happens quite often.

In one of my later studies, when I had already learned a fair bit from my mistakes and from kind colleagues, I had just about everything ready to take my first large mailing of something like 200 questionnaires to the local Post Office; everything was there and the return date had been printed on the documents so that it all had a most professional finish. Incidentally, I think it helps quite a lot to make all the material that is sent out look appealing; an attractive top sheet makes all the difference.

Well, what went wrong? The local Post Office would not accept the parcel as there was a threat of a postal strike. It had not yet begun but the officials did not want to have a large parcel 'stuck' in the system. I tried the General Post Office, also without success. The strike materialised and lasted 2 weeks. So by the time the parcels were eventually accepted, the date originally given for return of the questionnaires was no longer realistic, which meant having to alter, by hand, every single document which amounted to 400 alterations. The final appearance of the top sheet had to be sacrificed as there was not enough money available to reprint and rebind the material. In any case, it would have delayed the process even further and, even if money had been no problem, such an additional expense would not really have been justified.

Another time, when everything was ready for field work which entailed interviewing nursing staff in hospitals, we encountered a strike of ancillary workers. What did this have to do with our interviews? Everything. The nurses had to do ancillary work, and to spend time on research interviews was just about the lowest on their list of priorities. When the strike was over, a large number of nursing staff were due extra leave in lieu of days worked during the strike, so it was a whole month later before we could begin our interviews.

As a result of the delay my colleagues and I worked non-stop for a month; when the study's sponsors heard about it, they commented 'If we had known, you could have had some additional money for a temporary assistant.'

The third strike which upset my research plan was a rail strike which, in itself, would not have been too bad—after all one can get around by car. However, driving during a rail strike is no joke, especially when many petrol stations run out of petrol. At that time I was sorely tempted to replace my carefully constructed sample list by another, consisting of people who lived much closer. I am glad I held out and waited; I might have ruined the study and my reputation.

Not all delays and upheavals of the 'best-laid plans' are due to strikes. What do you do if your study involves the comparison of care on two different wards and suddenly, because of money having to be spent before the end of the financial year, it is decided to close one of the wards for redecorating? That decision put an end to one of my studies altogether. The administrator who made the decision was not in the least concerned about the research; it was not 'his' responsibility. Have you heard of the tale of the disappearing patient? Let me tell you. In the mid-1960s I was trying to find out if some surgical patients could be discharged from hospital earlier than had been the routine up to that time. Seemingly, many patients were kept in hospital only while waiting for their sutures or clips to be removed, a task which could be performed by the district nursing staff once the patients were home. We studied the records and, right enough, patient after patient was admitted for simple surgical procedures; within one month, according to our calculations, we should get enough patients, allowing for drop-outs, to make a meaningful comparison between an experimental group of 'early discharge' patients and a control group of 'routine discharge' patients.

We were all set, but the patients did not get admitted; we waited, the study period was extended and it took not 1 month but 3 to achieve the number we needed. One lady developed a stitch abscess after her surgery and, therefore, no longer fulfilled the criteria of 'normal recovery' but she was quite anxious to get home so I included her without saying anything to anyone. It was not worth it; my conscience gave me no peace at all and, fortunately, the patient moved out of our area and had to be dropped from the study anyway. I nearly cheated to get the numbers. In fact, I did, but was given the chance to get straight again.

This type of strange event, the disappearing patient, happens quite often. Stroke is a condition which, because of its frequency, has assumed an important place in the league table of morbidity in the elderly. Soon after a major stroke study was set up in Edinburgh, the incidence of the type of stroke we were interested in, appeared to drop and we were hard pressed to secure our planned number of patients. I could cite other incidents in studies I have been involved in and in those of other researchers.

Other well-made plans that were brutally destroyed related to a change in a specific surgical procedure which was being studied, a change in surgeon and a change in the data processing system which had been agreed. In all three cases, the research process was seriously hampered and urgent emergency decisions needed to be taken.

Data processing is worth an additional mention. First, I had to learn from my own bitter mistakes that the arrangements for data processing must be made at the very beginning of a study—probably in conjunction with the statistical advice. One has to book time which requires some kind of forecasting, and holdups, such as those I have mentioned, play havoc with even the most carefully calculated prediction. The other points about data processing are that the system may be changed without warning and that it is extremely expensive.

I had data on a computer in London after my move

to Edinburgh, data which I was still working on. For the first few months the systems in Edinburgh and London were compatible; then the changes came and I was in a ghastly dilemma. It made it necessary for me to cut the analysis of my data short which was a great pity; the alternative was a complete re-ordering of the material which, at that time, was out of question. Due to the expense of data-processing it is important to be quite sure what kind of analysis one needs and wants and to ensure that the data are really 'clean'; that means they have been checked for errors. Mistakes are costly, not only in money but also in time. One may have to wait in a long queue for a re-run. It is also a good idea not to be taken in by computer scientists, which means that one should try to acquire a basic knowledge of computer application for oneself. It was easy for me to be told that what I wanted in terms of an analysis could not be done; I believed it because I had too little knowledge to contradict.

I wrote in my jotter: 'Computer people are a bit like garage mechanics or watch repairers; they know that you don't know a lot and do what they like. I wish I had more knowledge to challenge them. I think all researchers should learn the rudiments of computer know-how; not the details, they should be left to the specialists, just the basics. If I had my life over again I'd make sure of that; it is too late now.'

Hindsight advice

1. Be prepared for strikes and other hold-ups and don't get too upset about them. Notify your sponsors immediately of

likely delays beyond your control; in fact, it is quite a good idea to notify them of any likely delay in the proposed time schedule.

2. Try to design your study in such a way that some slight adjustments are possible, should the need arise. For example, widen the initial criteria for inclusion in the study if at all possible, but do *not* slacken once the criteria have been agreed.

3. Make arrangements for data processing as soon as possible and make sure that your data are 'clean' before you pass them on.

4. Try to learn the basic principles of computer science, so that you know what the experts are talking about and so that you can tell them what you want.

   (If you cannot find a teacher, try your children or grandchildren!)

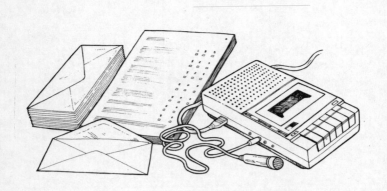

Five
Getting the information

In most of my early work, in fact in most of all my work, I used interviews, postal questionnaires and observation to get the information I wanted. In one study I asked nurses to complete a work diary.

I do wish that someone had told me that the information one gets is almost totally dependent on the way one asks for it. Moreover, if one really believes one gets at the truth, one may be sorely mistaken. Human beings can be extremely deceitful, either deliberately or unintentionally. They will tell you what they want you to know or what they think you want to hear and that is often suggested to them by the way the questions are asked.

Let me start with interviews: I used semi-structured interviewing schedules. They had some clear multiple choice type questions and some were open-ended, giving the respondents an opportunity to make additional comments or give answers which had not been anticipated. For example, I wanted to get the marital status of the district nurses and the question was: 'Are you single, married, divorced/separated, widowed?' Then, unless the answer was 'single' I proceeded to ask about children. One of the nurses remarked to me: 'I see you are leaving out a whole

37

chunk. Why is that?' I replied 'That section is all about children and you are single.' Without flinching she commented 'What makes you think that I can't have kids just because I'm single?' She was honest and outspoken. How many nurses would have offered this information so readily? I noted this incident down because it taught me that I had to be prepared for *all* eventualities and, therefore, one should always have a category called 'other' as a kind of safety net. A scribble which made me chuckle said that for the time being anyway male and female would cover all possibilities of sex, although 'who knows for how much longer?'

Reading about research interviewing in the few books which were available at that time, I realized that the wording of questions was important and could significantly influence the answer; I had already experienced this to be true. I had once asked nurses: 'In view of what we now know about the sterilization of equipment do you think that Method A is still safe?' It clearly provoked a negative answer. Fortunately, I noticed that in time, at least I was helped to notice it, and the question was changed to something like: 'Some people believe that equipment should be sterilized by Method A, others by Method B; which do you think is the safer of the two?' I cannot recall the precise words now but I hope that my example makes the point that questions can so easily be biased, that is they are more likely to get one answer than another. From this question I also learned that one must make provision for 'Don't know' or 'Not answered'. Respondents should be reassured that they can give a 'Don't know' answer and that they can also refuse to answer a certain question.

It is not only the wording of the questions which is important and which must remain static if a structured interviewing schedule is used. One cannot change the questions from one interview to the next for the reasons I have already referred to and for other reasons.

The other important point to remember, when interviews are used for getting information, is that facial expression and tone of voice can make an enormous difference to the way the question is answered. One of my questions was 'Why did you become a nurse?' In one of our teaching sessions, I watched and heard one of our hired interviewers, a non-nurse, asking a nurse respondent 'Why *did* you become a nurse?' The emphasis coupled with the frown on her face was enough to make the poor nurse quite apologetic about her career choice. Interviewing is a skill which must be learned.

Prompting or explaining are other ways which can influence the answer and one must be quite certain when, how and for what reasons one would allow a prompt. Again, I learned it the hard way: we were asking GPs how they felt about enrolled nurses caring for their patients. Some GPs asked what an enrolled nurse was; in my pilot study I left the explanation to the interviewer and asked her to write down how she had done it. One stated: 'An enrolled nurse is one who is not academic enough to pass the exams for state registration; her course is simpler and less academic'; another: 'the enrolled nurse's course is shorter and some young people just can't wait to get into a proper nursing job; I know an enrolled nurse who did that course because she wanted to keep nursing patients and not be pushed on.'

I looked at the answers given by the two GPs who had been given these explanations. It will not surprise anyone to know that the first said that he did not want enrolled nurses caring for his patients: in fact, he elaborated on his answer by remarking: 'I don't want a moron'; the other replied: 'Yes, I would like a nurse who is really interested in nursing rather than being academic.' The above comments relate to just two incidents from which one cannot generalize; I don't know if those GPs would have answered differently with different explanations and prompts. All I know *now* and, therefore, want to pass on, is that every respondent should receive exactly the same explanation or prompt. Otherwise one cannot tell if differences could be results of different prompts.

My last tale relating to interviews concerns ambiguity of questions. Readers may recognize the following incident because I have used it over and over again in my teaching. We were interviewing patients who had been asked to attend hospital outpatient departments for certain treatments such as the removal of sutures. The interview took place in the outpatient departments and one question was: 'How much does your return journey cost you?'

The question seemed straightforward enough and had already been answered without a problem by around 100 people. However, while I was personally interviewing a lady in a hospital on the south coast, she hesitated before answering this particular question and asked: 'You mean the bus back home from here, don't you?' I clearly remember feeling quite sick. She had misunderstood the question; my research colleagues and I had interpreted 'return journey' as the journey to the hospital and back home again; this dear lady had been taken to the hospital by her husband on his way to work and, therefore, she only thought in terms of paying her bus fare back home. It was an ambiguous and therefore a poor question and should have been changed before we began to interview people all over the country.

Of course, I alerted my colleagues and we decided to clarify the question for future interviews, but what were we to do with the answers we had already received? Could we assume that because no-one else had queried it, it had been interpreted in the way intended or could it be that people's answers depended on their own differing interpretation? To be quite honest, the temptation was to leave well alone and to assume that my lady was the only person who had doubts about the meaning of the question.

However, the problem niggled on and I felt uneasy about making such an unwarranted assumption. Several alternatives presented themselves; finally, it was decided to re-calculate all the expense figures given to us by asking the local nursing staff what the public transport costs for the 100 people already interviewed were likely to be. It seemed that the tempting initial assumption would have been justified as the figures proved right for both journeys—but, we could not have been sure. It was a mistake which was extremely tiresome to rectify; it took many hours of work. I think it was worth it, if only to teach us all an important lesson. At the time, the lady who had raised the question in the first instance did not endear herself to me—indeed I was almost angry with her. Hindsight makes me thankful to her.

In one study I asked nurses which, if any, professional journals they read, giving them the choice of the five most popular ones. To my amazement, they seemed to read the lot. Fortunately, my suspicious nature prevailed and I remembered that people will tell you what they would like you to hear. I abandoned the multiple choice element in the question and simply asked: 'Which, if any, professional journals do you read?' The answers changed radically and, apart from the regular one or two best known ones, the other three were hardly mentioned. Even the best known journals were mentioned by just a few of the respondents. Two of the journals, reported as being 'read regularly' in my exploratory study, never had a mention.

Self-completion questionnaires

I certainly did not get by unscathed in the use of this method of collecting information. I jotted down two painful experiences which I shall relate here but I had many more. The first incident is dated November 1968 and reads as follows: 'I thought people would be happier to give me their age by fitting it into an age group rather than telling me their actual age.'

So I had pre-determined groupings on the questionnaire:

18–30 1
30–40 2
40–50 3
50+ 4

People were instructed to circle the number opposite their age group. I had one questionnaire back which said 'I am celebrating my 30th birthday today, where do I belong?' What a sensible question! Of course, she could have fitted into two categories and that is extremely bad.* I should have known better, but how do you know if no-one tells you?' In the same survey one questionnaire was returned blank with a polite covering letter which said: I'm not quite 18, so I don't qualify; sorry!' I am glad I recorded those examples because now I would have found it hard to believe that I made such stupid mistakes.

Of course, there are other problems of ambiguity which apply to self-completion questionnaires, some of them even worse. I once asked a group of district nurses 'How many hours a week do you normally work?' It would be hard for me to explain now what *I* meant; it certainly was ambiguous; did I want paid hours or hours actually worked? Did I mean to have 'on call' hours included? What does 'normally' mean?

Observation

If anyone should think that observation is an easy method of collecting information, my experience suggests that this is far from true. As I mentioned in

*Age groupings should be mutually exclusive, e.g. 18–29, 30–39.

Chapter One, I wanted to observe district nurses to discover how they sterilized their equipment. Later, in another study, I wanted to know what nurses did and how much time they spent on their various activities. I started off with a blank piece of paper hoping, naively, to capture the information I wanted, using my own brand of shorthand. It did not take me long to find out the total impossibility of this approach although it helped me to design a more suitable form.

When my first day's observations were perused two weaknesses were suspected; first, most, if not all of my entries referred to the things I had expected to see; there was almost nothing unexpected, which appeared unlikely if not impossible; second, the difficulty, experienced during my recording and glaringly obvious in the completed sheets of paper (five sheets for one day!) the unwieldiness of my entries. There was no way in which one could disentangle the information and, because nurses appeared to perform more than one activity at the same time, it was impossible to decide on time spans. Take, for example, the task of 'washing a patient.' A nurse would go into the patient's kitchen to put the kettle on—not merely a matter of pressing a switch—in situations where water had to be heated on a kitchen range which quite often had to be lit in the first instance. While the water was heating she would search cupboards for clean linen. She would then bring the patient a bowl to encourage her—my entry referred to an old lady—to wash her own face, using this time to check that there was some food in the house. I hope I have made my point: when did 'washing a patient' start and finish?

I also recorded, or at least tried to record, what the nurse said to her elderly patient because I wanted to show the health teaching function of a district nurse. When I tried to analyse my day's entry I categorized a discussion about the lunch the old lady had eaten the day before as 'health teaching'; was I justified in doing this? Hindsight says 'no', because another observer may not have categorized it in this way.

Now I know that my first attempt at recording nursing activities lacked objectivity, validity and reliability. It lacked objectivity because I read into my observations what I wanted to see and hear; it lacked validity because I was not sure if I was really observing what I thought I was observing, such as health teaching; it lacked reliability because I could not be sure that anyone else would have made the same recording; in fact I was more sure that they would not.

My colleagues and I spent many weeks designing a better form and I am quite sure that this was far from foolproof; it was an improvement, but it could not overcome totally the difficulty of human limitations in observation of any kind. We were also grappling with the eternal problems of clear definitions. We had three observers and I wrote on one of the observation sheets which I kept: 'She seemed to call helping a patient to wash her own face 'general nursing care'. Mrs X called it "rehabilitation", while I called it "patient teaching". We really ought to have cleared all this up—too late now.'

Work diaries

As the observation of district nurses which includes a

great deal of travelling time is not only time-consuming and, therefore, expensive, but also liable to bias, introduced by observers and observed persons, I decided in a major national study to ask the nursing staff to keep diaries of their work. Easier and more reliable? Don't you believe it. Of course, the nurses had exactly the same problems that we had experienced as observers, namely, how do you draw the boundary between different activities and, how on earth do you get it all down on paper? Many problems were discussed with the nursing staff during the planning period and, eventually, we came up with a neat work record book which fitted easily into the outer pocket of the nurses' bags, in the hope that they would complete it after each visit or other activity and not to have to rely on the vagaries of memory. They were to fill it in for 7 days and then leave it at a collection point for the research team.

It became obvious that we had made several mistakes of which the following were the most annoying, at least according to my jotting of 15 years ago: 'Never trust nurses to fill in such a record immediately; they obviously didn't and we should have collected the books every day at least. Also why didn't we realize that the last week of March, which we had chosen for this exercise, was an atypical week, being the last week of the holiday year?' Some nurses were obviously far too busy to be conscientious over diary entries because they had to fill in for their colleagues on leave. Just to add to this particular problem, one nurse wrote on the first page of her diary: 'Don't think this is my normal work. Because I was told I had to fill this thing in, my pal took some of my work off me, as the writing took up a lot of my time.' Many entries didn't make any sense and I concluded: 'I think we should have done it for a 2 week period, 1 week gives a wrong impression.'

However, taking the survey as a whole and linking the work diary with the interviews which were part of the study, we managed to get some useful results and the overall analysis demonstrated findings which certainly had face validity—they looked right and formed a useful basis for discussion.

There are many other methods for collecting information; I have discussed three only because I used them more frequently and I wrote notes about them.

Hindsight advice

All methods of collecting information from human beings have inherent difficulties and one must choose the most suitable for the purpose.

1. Questions, whether they are part of an interviewing schedule or a self-administered questionnaire, must be unambiguous, mutually exclusive and make provision for all possible answers. They must be carefully tested before their final use.
2. If explanations or prompts must be given they should be standardized.
3. Interviews for research purposes require special skills which must be learned and interviewers should be trained.
4. If respondents are offered 'acceptable' answers they are likely to choose them whether they are true or not.
5. In the choice of a particular time period for the collection

of information advice should be sought concerning its suitability. It is worth noting, however, that people nearly always find reasons why a suggested time is not suitable.

6. Self-completion records should be collected as soon as possible after their expected completion; obvious queries and errors could then be clarified.

7. If only part of a work force has been selected as a sample of people to help with a time-consuming exercise such as the completion of a work diary, the possibility of distortion of the work should be considered; there are ways around it!

8. The period over which the completion of a diary or similar recording is requested should be sufficiently long to allow a reasonable coverage of the full range of work, including getting used to the record keeping; however, it must not be so long that it generates annoyance, boredom and diminishing returns in terms of conscientiousness.

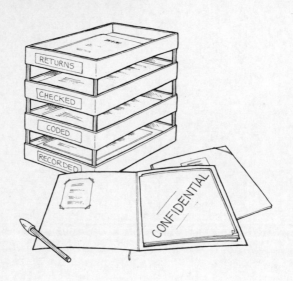

Six
More hazards of field work

An important part of field work is the mechanics of it all. Somehow one has to get self-completion forms, if these are being used, to the right respondents; one has to identify the respondent without putting a name on any of the forms, one has to record the return of completed (or uncompleted) forms and one has to make some provision for reminder letters if these are to be sent. If the specific project also includes interviews and perhaps data sheets for the extraction of information from records, the amount of paper which has to be ordered and taken care of can be substantial.

In one of my studies, we used three different data collection sheets (research tools) for nurses, two different types of sheets for GPs and an interviewing schedule for nursing administrators. Eventually they were all to be linked. They were ordered according to geographical region and, of course, each potential respondent had a unique identification code number. The code number had five digits: one for the region, one for the type of respondent and three for the serial number, allowing for as many as 999 respondents. The self-completion forms for GPs and nurses consisted of several sheets of paper each, stapled together. The unique number was clearly printed on the top sheet and each set of forms was accompanied by a covering letter addressing the person by name, asking for their co-operation and assuring them of confidentiality as well as anonymity.

I would like to share with you three risk points and one bad mistake.

First, the risk points: We sent a personal letter, addressing the person by name and promising anonymity. Most of our respondents accepted it all without question. However, two people, one GP and one nurse wrote extremely upset letters and another GP telephoned in a rage. The reason for their concern was the apparent inconsistency between addressing them by name, giving them a number and promising them anonymity. The doctor on the telephone was angry and I kept the gist of his complaint for teaching purposes. He said something like: 'How dare you think that I'm such an idiot as not to link my name with your impressive looking magic number; if you are as impertinent as that I will certainly not fill the... form in. Get lost!' Down went the telephone and I was shattered. The letters had a similar content but their tone was a little more gentle and they asked for reassurance that the number was not just a code for their name. Of course, it was; how else could we tell who returned their forms, how else could we send reminder letters? I was angry, upset and bewildered.

What had gone wrong? How could we save the situation? Why didn't somebody tell me what I should have done? It seemed obvious that we had not given enough information about the exact meaning of confidentiality and anonymity in the context of research. The three people who had voiced their concern deserved a letter of apology and explanation, but what about the others? I had no hesitation in writing a *polite* letter to the irate GP assuring him that I realized that he would see the connection between name and number but that the code list linking the two was locked away in our research safe and once the forms were completed (expressing my sincere hope that he would reconsider his initial decision), the list would be destroyed; it would only be used to check the returns. I am happy to relate that he did co-operate and with his completed form he sent an apologetic letter. I wrote to the other two people giving them the same explanation; of course, they could not be reassured that there was no link between number and name. I thanked them both for their letters and all was well. They also participated.

The question 'What about the others?' remained unanswered. Having been told and convinced that all respondents in a research project should be given exactly the same information as their answers might be influenced by it, I decided to write the same letter to them all, explaining the meaning of these two perplexing terms 'confidentiality' and 'anonymity'. I told them that confidentiality meant that no names would be mentioned in any report and that their information would be used only for the purpose of this particular research project. I explained anonymity and the use of the number as indicated above. Five people wrote in answer to my letter telling me that I had got them worried and they would rather not participate; one, believe it or not, wrote to say that there was no point in going to all that trouble if nobody knew that it was he who held such strong views; therefore, he would not bother, he had not thought about it before. It really is hard to win!

The second risk point concerned the way the envelopes to the respondent and the enclosed reply envelopes were addressed and stamped. We used brown manilla envelopes, addressed them to the work place and franked them; the reply envelopes were stamped. I would not do any of these things again; franked brown manilla envelopes are not opened with great glee and, I knew from other instances, that in some GP practices such mail may never ever reach the GP personally. I also know that some people use stamped envelopes for other purposes. It may have happened in this study; I don't know I refer to it as a risk point rather than a serious mistake because we had a response rate of over 80% which, for a study of this sort, was encouraging. It could have been a disaster.

The third extremely risky and careless part of that large postal study was the inadequate preparation for the recording of returns and the dates of reminder letters. Certainly, a special book had been prepared for the purpose but it was not completed conscientiously enough. Fortunately, the number of required reminder letters and duplicate questionnaires was minimal—but I confess much more due to good fortune than to meticulous preparation.

The extremely severe mistake was the fact that we printed the identification number on the top sheet of the set of papers only. It was a mistake for two reasons; in the first place, the stapling was not secure enough to ensure that the forms would not come apart during the tedious process of checking and coding which entailed extensive manual handling. Many did and we had to put them together by matching the handwriting—an enormously time-consuming and risky business. Secondly, it would have been possible to send single pages to be code-punched thus saving a great deal of time. I had not even identified those pages which obviously required a new computer card and those numbers had to be laboriously added later, using five precious columns which had been reserved for other information in our carefully constructed coding instructions. I realize that modern processing techniques may render this specific instance irrelevant but it epitomizes many serious errors which could be avoided if the appropriate knowledge were freely available. At that time it was not and it is possible that the present day scene may be riddled with other hazards which future generations of researchers need to be warned about.

The process between checking completed questionnaires and making them computer-ready is laborious; all the information which is to be computerized has to be transferred to numbers, the process of coding already referred to. Sensible and unambiguous coding instructions are absolutely crucial, especially if several persons are involved in coding. It would be fairly easy for me to write a book just on the problems of coding and the many lessons I learned and still have to learn from mistakes that I and/or members of my research teams made. In my naivety it had not occurred to me that a coder might actually change the coding because she thought the respondent could not have meant what had been clearly written, but it happened. When I saw the alteration on a spot check I asked the coder and she said: 'Well I happen to know that GP and he must have misunderstood the question.'

She committed two cardinal sins; first, she used the identification code in the interpretation of the information (although she insisted that she recognized the handwriting which is not much better) and, second, she made an alteration based on her own ideas and judgement. The alteration was, of course, reversed to the original and that coder was given another batch of forms. I also went through all her completed coding work looking for similar breaches of the basic research rules; I found none—fortunately for us both.

The biggest coding problems I found I had to cope with concerned open-ended material; the many, many different answers and shades of answers one got were not easily handled. Decisions had to be made about putting some answers together although they were not identical or having so many different codes that one could not use them in the analysis anyway. I am sure that I made many more mistakes than I even know about. Do such comments made by patients as 'I can't tell you how glad I was to get home' and 'Well, under the circumstances I was really glad to get home' mean the same or don't they? Who knows? What about 'I thought I would like district nursing'? Does it mean she thought she would and didn't, or she thought she would and did?

Questions, answers and coding of the answers all play tricks—so beware!

Hindsight advice

1. Make quite certain that letters and self-completion forms are clear and that the ethical principles of confidentiality and anonymity, where promised, are explained and respected.
2. In a postal survey use white stamped envelopes wherever possible; it is also a good idea to mark the envelope 'Personal', so that it does not get opened by anyone else.
3. Use 'Freepost' addressed envelopes for the replies: they cannot be used for any other purpose. (At my time they were not available.)
4. Put the identification number on each sheet in a set of forms and staple them securely in more than one place; binding may be better still.
5. Keep open-ended questions to a minimum; they are often best used for anecdotal purposes only, rather than for coding; one can so easily add 'apples and oranges' together making them one.
6. Carefully check the coding process; genuine mistakes can easily be made and obvious errors can be corrected. It is not allowed to tamper for any reason whatever with answers given by respondents. Such alterations offend the most fundamental research rule.

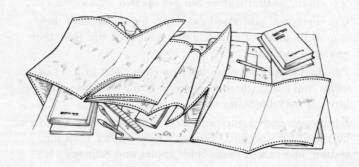

Seven
Making sense of it all

The information obtained by a gamut of methods, some more appropriate than others, had to be disentangled and made some sense of; it had to be interpreted.

I found this stage to be one of the most difficult in the whole research process. My first experience in handling computer print-out, which occurred in 1966, I have related many times, but, because it taught me important lessons, it is worth mentioning in the context of my other many woes and follies. At that time, computers were really quite a novelty, especially in nursing research. I had little idea of what they could or could not do, hence my hindsight advice at the end of Chapter Four, and I had even less idea of what a computer print-out looked like.

Because I was, at that time, not working in an organization which had its own data processing facilities, I was advised to approach a university department which accepted outside work on a contract basis. This I did, although it took a long time to agree on appropriate terms especially as I was working within a limited budget.

Fortunately, help came eventually, although rather late and in a small measure. When I took possession of my first 'print-out' I was close to fainting point; it was delivered in the form of a huge roll of paper, resembling stair carpet for a six storey mansion. What was I to do with it? It was even difficult to unfold its mystery in terms of unrolling the extremely heavy mass of paper.

With some effort I secured it firmly by means of a cupboard on the top floor of the building I was working in and treated it like stair carpet; that is, I unrolled it slowly and clumsily down three flights of stairs, having put a notice in the front entrance hall, asking people to use the lift as the stairs were 'temporarily out of bounds'. It was then a matter of getting down on my hands and knees, starting from the ground floor and working my way up just to read what the paper carpet contained. To my joy and relief I eventually found some lines with page numbers, obviously indicators that one could cut the monster at those points, thereby making it manageable. Now, 20 years later, computer output reaches us in a much more acceptable form, almost ready for immediate consumption.

Computer language seemed to have few words and millions of figures, many of which I did not understand. I was used to communication between humans and suddenly to have to hold a sensible conversation with a machine was perplexing, to say the least. 'Totals' was a term I knew (surprise!) but 'missing cases' puzzled me, especially as the missing cases seemed to exceed the totals quite often. If cases are missing how can you total them? Yes, I was as naive as that.

What the computer had provided for me at that time was a complete straight count of all the variables in my study and there were hundreds of them which seemed like billions. Having asked too many questions in the first instance certainly did not help. I was suffocating in my own data some of which were not only irrelevant but literally useless.

I had data for GPs, data for district nurses, data for nursing administrators and everything about all of them had been carefully counted, including the 'missing cases'. I had GPs under the age of 30 years and I had some who were 60 and over. My first urge was to see if my hunch that older GPs were not as keen on working as partners with nurses as younger ones was true. Alas, it did not look like it all. A larger number of the 'over 60s' expressed enthusiastic views about the possibility of working more closely with their nursing colleagues than the number of those who were under the age of 30. I was disappointed; remember I said, at the end of Chapter Two that, if one sets out to prove a point one may be disappointed. In fact, I was devastated because I had already mentally seen the headlines in the nursing journals 'New report finds older GPs are against district nurses'. Then, some of my wiser colleagues looked at the data and the picture changed. I had not seen that there were many more older GPs than younger ones and, therefore, the much smaller number of 'under 30s' represented a larger percentage of the total than that of the older group.

I was led on to look at percentages; ah, the computer print-out said that 95% of GPs over the age of 65 thought that . . . ; it does not really matter what they thought, what does matter is the fact that 95% of that group amounted to only 1.4 GP and what can one make of that? So, were older GPs less likely than younger ones to have a desire to work more closely with district nurses? In percentage terms it began to look like it but, alas, the statistician said that the difference was not 'statistically significant'. Therefore, I knew from my beginners' statistics classes, the difference could have been due to chance. What a pity!

What about the district nurses? I had many more of them in my study, and, therefore some comparisons between them were more likely to be statistically significant. Three cheers! Married nurses spent significantly more time teaching patients' relatives than single ones. I started writing: 'Married nurses are used to having to think of preparing meals for their families and to making their husband and children less dependent on them; therefore, married nurses are more alert to teaching responsibilities than single ones; they also appreciate the cost of things more and, therefore, give better advice on housekeeping generally.' How dared I make such statements from my simple straight counts? My jotting says: 'Mr X told me that I am just using my fantasy and not my data and that I am reading into the figures far more than I am allowed to.' Of course, Mr X was totally right. All I had was counts and no support at all for any speculation on the reasons for those counts. I was advised to ask the computer for further, slightly more sophisticated, analyses, such as two-way tables, significance tests and correlation coefficients, hardly sophisticated by present standards but extremely advanced for me at that time. To my dismay the computer was 'out of commission' for 2 whole weeks and then had to cope with a backlog of work.

Believe me, even now such things happen with monotonous regularity!

I set to, calculating all those things with the aid of a slide rule which was extremely tedious, but amazingly instructive. It also helped me later when I had to take my statistics examination where we were only allowed slide rules.

I came up with 'fascinating' findings, for example, I had a correlation coefficient of $+0.90$ between the distances from a nurse's base to her district and the time she took for travelling—hardly a world-shaking research finding though. That sort of thing happened because I had *everything* in my study tested against *everything*; it was a total waste of time and precious money. 'Why didn't someone advise me to be much more selective?'

I had asked the district nurse to add any comments or suggestions at the end of the questionnaire; more older ones than younger ones did so. My draft report stated: 'Younger nurses are clearly less interested than older ones in their profession; they cannot even be bothered to make comments.'

It soon came out of my report; I had no right at all to say it.

My jotting says: 'It is probably best just to write down your findings and let people make their own deduction from them.' This has proved to be true, at least most of the time and research methods' books which have become available since my feeble attempts, seem to support it. Clearly, one cannot make any statement about cause and effect simply because two figures show a high positive correlation with each other. However, having said that, I discovered that no interpretation at all was not too helpful either. People kept writing and asking what it all meant and the administrators, particularly, said 'lots of tables but so what'?'.

I then decided to present the data as they were, but to write a separate part giving possible interpretations.

My note says: 'People can't quarrel with my findings but they have a right to read them in a different way from my own.'

Hindsight advice

1. Make yourself reasonably familiar with the expected format of your data; it will prevent a shock.
2. Be selective in the data to be counted, tabulated and calculated. Remember that the computer is a moron and depends on your commonsense.
3. Make a clear distinction between the research findings—pure and not tampered with—and your personal speculations about what they *may* mean.
4. Make sure that you understand the meaning of any statistical tests which you are asking the computer to calculate for you.
5. Do not infer causal relationships between findings obtained from a descriptive study; such inferences are rarely, if ever, justified.

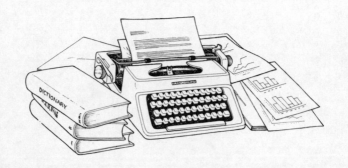

Eight

Getting the findings across

In the preceding chapter I mentioned the above, somewhat scathing comment 'so what?' in relation to the interpretation of research data, of figures, tables, graphs etc. I soon discovered that the production of large amounts of data in whatever form was not the end of my problems. Somehow they had to be communicated to 'whoever'. The 'whoever' is a significant variable in this communication process because different people have different expectations and also different levels of understanding. Moreover, they have different ideas about the use to which the research findings might be put.

My early work was requested by my employing organization and a report of it had to be presented to a committee consisting of mainly lay and a few professional members. One or two represented academic establishments. I was told that my report should be no more than 20–30 pages long; no-one would be interested or have time to read through a longer document. It seemed to me that the best way to get a great deal of information into the fewest possible pages was to produce many tables which saved words.

So, my first draft report had three parts; the first part said why the research project had been undertaken

and included polite thank you's to dozens of people
who had contributed in one way or another; in other
words, the acknowledgements which proved to be an
absolute 'must' for courtesy and for diplomatic reasons.
The second part consisted of something like 60 tables
and a few figures, such as histograms and pie-charts,
just to ring the changes. In the final part I picked out
one or two of the findings which I wanted the
committee to know about. The usual reference list
followed; fortunately, as I explained in Chapter One it
was a very short list indeed because not much research
had been found in this particular field.

The report was duly circulated and put on the
agenda for the next meeting of the committee. Oh dear!
My notes say: 'What a lot of queer people! Do they
really know what they want and how can I please them
all in 30 pages?' What had happened was that some
members said that they did not understand the tables;
others did not believe the tables and thought that I
must have 'got it wrong'. The academics told me that
results of research had no validity unless the reader
knew how they had been obtained; in other words, they
wanted the method of the study included. Still others
and also some of the above critics wanted, above all,
recommendations. I remember feeling and, obviously
looking, extremely down-hearted until somebody said:
'Don't feel that we are negative about your work. It's
fine. It only needs ...'

'It only needs ...' I had run out of time and
available finance. The amendments referred to as 'only'
would not merely take an enormous amount of
additional work and certainly a complete re-typing, but

some were obviously impossible to comply with. For example, I did not feel that my small study warranted definite recommendations other than more research. With a great deal of midnight oil and amateur typing I managed to arrive at an acceptable compromise—less tables, a little more explanatory narrative and inclusion of the method, thereby enabling readers to judge the authenticity of the results. The report finally passed the test and everyone was happy; my extreme exhaustion was not a relevant variable in that situation! Some of the agony could certainly have been avoided.

My friends in the Nursing Research Discussion Group encouraged me to send my report to one of the nursing journals for publication. At that time we were really short of such material but, of course, we did not know whether nurse readers would be interested. I duly sent a manuscript to two journals at the same time—on the assumption that one, at least, would reject it. To my great amazement, both showed interest although both wanted different amendments in terms of length and in terms of content. One wanted me to retain the section 'methodology', the other did not; so I clinched a contract with the former.

Then I got into very hot water because my employers, unbeknown to me at the time of submitting my manuscript to the journals, decided to publish the whole report themselves without an author's name. After all, I had done the work in my working time so it was a report by the organization, not by me. Fair enough, but my manuscripts had gone off with my name and I was truly in a cleft stick having offended ethical conventions regarding copyright and publishing in general. It was made abundantly clear to me that one does *not* send the same manuscript to two journals and that one cannot have the same manuscript published under one's own name as would be published by someone else, though without an author's name.

The whole affair was unpleasant and unnecessary. Ignorance of what my employers had in mind did not release me from basic ethical and legal principles, and I had to withdraw my accepted manuscript from the journal. My rather depressed note at the time of my encounter with my employers says: 'I wonder how people can find a book that has no author.' (in this case the organization was author *and* publisher). I had some cause for concern, and, if I had been as sure then as I am now, I would have insisted.

Another, somewhat similar, mistake relating to publishing was made by me in connection with a multiple authorship report. I had not realized the convention of putting the main author first or, if there is no main author, to use alphabetical ordering of names. In this particular instance I lost out because, although I was main author, my name was not first in the alphabet; it reduced me to being referred to as 'et al' ever after, when this particular article was quoted. It did not really matter but it could have done, and I wish somebody had told me.

There is a great deal to be learned about submitting manuscripts and it can be done more painlessly than through mistakes or misconceptions. One of my publishers explained to me the need to give extremely careful consideration to the number of words and to their length—each word costs money and a longer word is not necessarily better than a shorter one. It was he who pointed out to me that a research project can *not* have a 'methodology' but only a 'method'. Methodology means the science of methods; just compare it with the many other 'ologies'; I wasted the precious space of five letters in addition to making a laughing stock of myself. I note now, many many years later, that other people should remember this also.

Although I made many mistakes in the presentation of my data my notes on them are rather sparse. One instance was recorded in some detail and, therefore, it must have caused me some concern at the time.

In one of my analyses, I had 45% of GPs giving a positive answer to a question about working with nurses in an 'attachment' situation and 45% answered the question negatively; the remaining 10% gave 'don't know' or inadequate answers. My jotting reads: 'Trust the Press to distort things. Here we are, the headline to my report says: *"GPs don't want to work with nurses" says new research report.* 'But I had never written that; what I had written was: 'In spite of the obvious advantages of working alongside nursing staff half the GPs did not want such an arrangement.' Looking at that report again I realized that it was as much my fault as the Journal's to create such a biased headline.

Two bad mistakes: don't link your own ideas with findings *and* give the full story and not half of it; people take in the half you tell them and not the other half. If I had written 'half the GPs liked the idea of working with nurses' the headlines might have presented the opposite view—simply because that was the part of the information given. What I should have done, I think, was to present the results in table form and either leave the message there or say something like 'as can be seen in Table X the GPs were equally divided in their views about whether they wanted to work with nurses or not.'

I realize that the instance I relate is possibly a rare coincidence; it is, however, representative of many similar types of data presentations which, by their incompleteness, may be perceived and interpreted in a distorted manner. What I learned from it was that a research report may be biased through what one *omits* to say, either deliberately or accidentally. Deliberate omission is unforgiveable and shows lack of integrity; accidental omission can be guarded against by special care and by getting someone else to look at the data *and* their presentation.

The other mistake which I recorded and which I have talked about ad nauseam ever since, related to the use of jargon which is incomprehensible to the people with whom we want to communicate. My note mentions two terms which had obviously given me problems: the first is 'postulating that my working hypothesis would be supported ...'; the second 'randomized controlled trial'. I could now think of better examples to make my point but will use those I recorded at the time. What I wrote was: 'a nurse asked me what "postulating" and "working hypothesis" meant and I think I could have said it in a much simpler way; too late now.' In the second case I noted: 'X told me today that I am just showing off by using fancy terms; It's upsetting because I thought X liked my work; she pointed out that no nurse can be expected to know what 'r.c.t.' (I had even abbreviated it just to add insult to injury) means. Well, I can't think of another term, but, perhaps I should have explained it. Whatever made me use such an abbreviation—I keep telling others not to do it.'

Hindsight advice

1. Unless research findings are published, they are of no use to anyone.
2. When submitting manuscripts, consider the target readership in the selection of the most suitable publication medium.
3. Do not send the same manuscript to more than one journal at the same time because each spends time and money on arriving at its decision.
4. If you are a joint author with others decide early on which way the authors should be listed.
5. Remember that what you do *not* say in a report may be as, if not more, important than what you do say. No-one will know but your conscience and integrity may suffer!
6. Use plain simple language whenever possible; if technical terminology is necessary—and it often is—explain it; a glossary of terms may be useful.
7. Try not to use abbreviations; if you do, give the full terms at least once.
8. Most research requires the help of several people; don't forget to acknowledge their help, not least any source of financial support and your research 'subjects' who because of anonymity, you may not be able to mention by name.

Epilogue

In the preface I stated the purpose of this small book; whether it has been achieved remains to be seen.

The hazards and mistakes represented by the eight chapters cover merely the tip of the iceberg of the number of things which can so easily go wrong in research. However, one learns from mistakes and they form an important part in the process of acquiring a measure of competence. Even if my hindsight advice should help some people to avoid just a few mistakes, there are still enough left from which learning is possible. Mistakes and misconceptions will, no doubt, continue; as far as I know, the perfect piece of research still remains to be done. It is my view, again formed through hindsight, that one of the most valuable parts of one's life is the opportunity for continual learning.

It must also be noted that my experiences cover early, mainly descriptive and quantitative studies only. Historical, philosophical, qualitative research and other approaches to exploring the universe pose many other problems. I have decided to close this epilogue by a brief, oversimplified summary of my hindsight advice, ordering it as closely as possible in the logical sequence of the research process.

Summary

1. Persist in questioning assumptions and routines but realize that not all questions are researchable, at least not in their original form.
2. Remember always that research requires its own specialized knowledge and skills; seek appropriate advice; it is more freely available than you may think.
3. Observe the code of ethics relating to research; if you need help, your professional organization should be able to give it—in the U.K., the Royal College of Nursing certainly would.
4. Create or join a group of other interested people; uninhibited discussion is supportive and helps in clarifying thinking.
5. If you are seeking financial support, get help in preparing your application.
6. Think about every stage of your planned project well in advance; get early statistical advice and explore the available data processing system. Set realistic time targets.
7. Examine your motives for doing the research; watch for possible biases; if you feel you cannot totally avoid them (which is virtually impossible anyway), declare them openly.
8. Undertake a careful search of the literature; if you find a large library daunting, ask for advice.
9. Make clear entries of the relevant literature, preferably on index cards; record all relevant information to enable you and others to locate it easily.

10. Choose the design, method and data collection tools appropriate for your particular research question.

11. Take great care in the design of your data collection tools; questionnaire design is difficult; it is equally, if not more, difficult to design simple forms which can capture observational data.

12. Be sure to undertake a thorough pilot study and analyse its results; write a report of it and draw up dummy tables.

13. Research interviewing requires special skills; it is *unlike* interviewing for the assessment of patients or for the selection of staff.

14. If coding is required compile clear unambiguous coding instructions and do not tamper with the original answers because they 'look wrong'.

15. Study your raw data carefully before giving computing instructions; it will help you in being selective in your requests.

16. Give great care to the presentation of your material at the end of all the hard work. The format may depend on your target readers; initially, these may be your sponsors; consider their wishes.

17. Consider the balance between numbers and words; both have their purpose.

18. Do *not* confuse research findings with their interpretation.

19. Make sure that any recommendations you want to make, arise from your findings and not from the bee in your bonnet.

20. Avoid extravagant and obtuse language. Where technical terminology is appropriate use it, but

provide an explanation if your target readers cannot be expected to have it in their vocabulary. Avoid abbreviations where possible.

21. Be honest in your presentation and own up to mistakes which may alter the use of the research.

22. If appropriate, explore the speedy publication of your work so that your colleagues may have the benefit of it. Consult publishers/editors of books and journals for advice regarding authorship, copyright, etc.

23. Check your list of references carefully; remember that its purpose is to help your readers to find the work you quoted.

24. Do not expect to 'change the world' by your research—you won't!

25. Be prepared for people to question your work, to criticize it and to pull it to pieces; it is all part of the exercise and *can* be extremely helpful.

Conclusion

It is my belief that a successful researcher requires at least five attributes and I do *not* imply that I have them; but neither do I claim success!

They are:

1. Curiosity
2. Competence
3. Integrity
4. Commonsense
5. Sense of humour.

I further believe that the first two of those attributes

can be acquired; the last three are gifts—three great gifts, the greatest of which is integrity.

In spite of all its hazards and problems, to be involved in research is a wonderful experience. Don't be put off but enjoy it!

Bibliography

Introduction

No book, however excellent, can adequately substitute practical experience as a 'research apprentice' or as a 'supervised research student' in providing a suitable preparation for independent research activity. Conversely, practical experience alone is not adequate either; it is important to obtain a wider picture of research issues and methods than one's individual experience can offer. Recourse to suitable literature might have saved me from some of my mistakes and misconceptions. As a 'research apprentice' one has a role model and as a 'supervised research student' one has a supervisor. My problem was that, during the early years of my research career, I had neither and, therefore, I lacked adequate guidance and direction in the use of the sparse literature which was available at the time.

When I decided to include a brief bibliography I considered ordering it in the logical sequence of the research process. The book edited by Cormack (1984) has done much of this work for me. I have arranged the literature from general to the more specific topics and have ignored its chronological or alphabetical order.

81

Five points need to be made in relation to this bibliography:

1. It represents a small selection of basic reference material dealing with the generic topic of research applicable to the study of nursing; it does not include texts on statistics.

2. It includes books, book chapters and booklets only. Journal articles are omitted, not because they are not important, but because they are too numerous.

3. The selection of books and the annotations are, of necessity, personal and subjective; other researchers are likely to have made a different selection and assessment.

4. A deliberate attempt has been made to include British and North American material. On both sides of the Atlantic and, indeed, in many other parts of the world, important contributions to the topic of nursing research have originated. Nurse researchers should resolve more fervently to adopt an international approach to their reading.

5. Each book cited has its own list of references which will take the reader further. To follow a reference list is a little like an obstacle race or an adventure trip; it is hard work but exciting and one wins eventually.

General issues

Smith J F 1981 Nursing science in nursing practice. Butterworths, London
Although this book is not directly relevant to research methodology it demonstrates that the subject matter of nursing is amenable to research.

McFarlane J K 1970 The proper study of the nurse. Royal College of Nursing, London
In presenting an account of the first two years of the Royal College of Nursing research project 'The study of nursing care', the author suggests a variety of approaches for the systematic study of nurses and nursing.

Downs F S, Fleming J W 1979 Issues in nursing research. Appleton Century Crofts, New York
The seven chapters cover important issues from the historical perspective to the future of nursing research. It touches on educational, ethical and theoretical aspects.

Simpson, M 1981 Issues in nursing research. In: Hockey L (ed) Current issues in nursing. Churchill Livingstone, Edinburgh
The author depicts the British scene of nursing research; she raises questions about the education of researchers, about financial support, about long term planning and many others.

Royal College of Nursing of the United Kingdom 1977 Ethics related to research in nursing. Royal College of Nursing, London
A small booklet setting out ethical guidelines for nursing research and representing the professional code relating to it.

Clark J M, Hockey, L 1979 Research for nursing—a guide for the enquiring nurse. HM & M Publishers, London

This small book is intended to introduce nurses to the meaning and potential of research. A selection of easily accessible research reports is used to demonstrate how the researchers tackled specific questions, which research designs and methods they used and what the implications of their findings might be for nursing. It includes a chapter on research training and research careers and discusses research as a change agent.

Basic tests on general research methodology

Cormack D F S 1984 The research process in nursing. Blackwell Scientific, London
As alluded to above, the editor of this helpful volume arranged the material in order of the process which has to be followed in the pursuit of research. It begins with the nature and purpose of research and ends, constructively, with four chapters on the application of nursing research. It includes some of the most commonly used research approaches.

Notter L E 1974 Essentials of nursing research. Springer, New York
Evidenced by various reprints, this small volume has met the basic needs of many beginning nurse researchers. It is an elementary text and includes a useful glossary of terms. Its examples and references are exclusively American.

Brink P J Wood, M J 1978 Basic steps in planning research. Wadsworth, Belmont, USA

The authors state clearly that they have provided a book which deals solely with the beginning phase of the research—the plan; as such it has some usefulness. A glossary of terms and suggestions for the future are helpful additions. It is exclusively American in its examples and references.

Fox D J 1977 Fundamentals of research in nursing. Appleton Century Crofts, New York

Treece E W, Treece J W Jr 1982 edition Elements of research in nursing. Mosby, Missouri

Both the above books are useful general textbooks covering the principles of research methodology and some basic statistics. In my view they are roughly equal in the level of sophistication although the publication by Treece & Treece is more comprehensive and, by virtue of its further editions, more up to date.

Polit P, Hungler B 1978 Nursing research. Lippincott, New York
An extremely comprehensive book, covering most aspects of general research topics, which was unknown to me until I visited a Canadian University in 1983 where it was widely used as standard reference text.

Seaman C H, Verhonick P J 1982 Research methods for undergraduate students in nursing. Appleton Century Crofts, New York
This is an enlarged and improved second edition of a

text published in 1978. It takes the reader through the research process at a basic level. Some useful technical details such as questionnaire lay-out and coding devices are included; in showing a questionnaire format, a tick $(\sqrt{})$ is advised as a check mark, a method which I warned against in Chapter 2.

The bibliography is comprehensive within the constraints of being American only.

Some specific research topics

Hoinville G, Jowell R 1977 Survey research practice. Heinemann Educational, London

Abramson J H 1974 Survey methods in community medicine. Churchill Livingstone, Edinburgh

Although neither of the above two books deals specifically with nursing both are important contributions to survey methods and have a relevant application to nursing. Both volumes are useful for nurses; Hoinville & Jowell, along with their associate authors, write within a framework of the social sciences whilst Abramson provides a guide for the design of studies concerned with health and disease.

Campbell D T, Stanley J C 1963 Experimental and quasi-experimental designs for research. Rand McNally, Chicago.

Although this book was published well over 20 years ago it is still the 'classic' on experimental design. It is not specific to nursing but the material can be and has been applied to nursing. Anyone planning an experimental study should consult this text.

Oppenheim A N 1966 Questionnaire design and attitude measurement. Heinemann, London
This book, reprinted several times, has remained a classic on the topic of its title. I found its section on attitudes, definitions, statements and measurements, particularly helpful.

Bennet A E, Ritchie K 1975 Questionnaires in medicine. Oxford University Press for the Nuffield Provincial Hospitals Trust, Oxford
The authors draw heavily on Oppenheim's publication but apply the principles to the field of health care. It includes helpful examples which are relevant for many nursing projects.

Glaser, B, Strauss A L 1967 The discovery of grounded theory: strategies for qualitative research. Aldine, Chicago
This is a seminal work in the field of qualitative research and should be consulted by anyone planning such an approach.

Burgess R G (ed) 1982 Field research: a source book and field manual. (Allen & Unwin, London
The specific aims of this comprehensive volume are stated to be:

to indicate the diverse approaches involved in doing field research to examine a range of research techniques that have been used in field research

to examine the problems that arise in the course of doing field research and the ways these problems have been handled by experienced field researchers

The book makes a most important contribution to research methodology by demonstrating how qualitative research can be scientifically credible.

Isaac S, Michael W B 1971 Handbook in research and evaluation. Edits Publishers, Sandiego, USA

The fact that this book had its 13th reprinting in 1980 indicates its appeal. It is referred to as a collection of principles, methods and strategies useful in the planning, design and evaluation of studies in education and the behavioural sciences. It includes a comprehensive overview of research designs, including historical research and action research. Its final chapter deals with evaluation criteria applied to a range of different problems. Statistical texts are deliberately omitted from this bibliography but a useful chapter on statistical techniques can be found in Isaac's volume.

By the time this book is published many more useful research texts are likely to be available. In the series 'Recent Advances in Nursing', published by Churchill Livingstone, a volume on Nursing Research Methodology has been initiated.

In addition to the literature on general research issues there is a rapidly increasing amount of specialised material available—specialised in terms of research strategies and methods and specialised also in terms of the topic being researched.

Indexes and bibliographies are indispensable guides to the literature.

Librarians are extremely helpful allies and almost always enjoy being consulted.

Whether involved in research or not, reading is every nurse's professional responsibility, at least in my view. I know that it is not always easy to make time for it but I also know that time spent on reading is always well worthwhile. It opens up new lines of thought and helps us to retain a healthy professional and academic curiosity. Reading aids learning and learning is one of the most exciting and rewarding activities which can and should be pursued throughout life.

Knowledge begets knowledge and there is no end.